BRAIN-BOOSTING RECIPES COOKBOOK FOR COGNITIVE WELLNESS

Nourish Your Mind, Fuel Your Potential

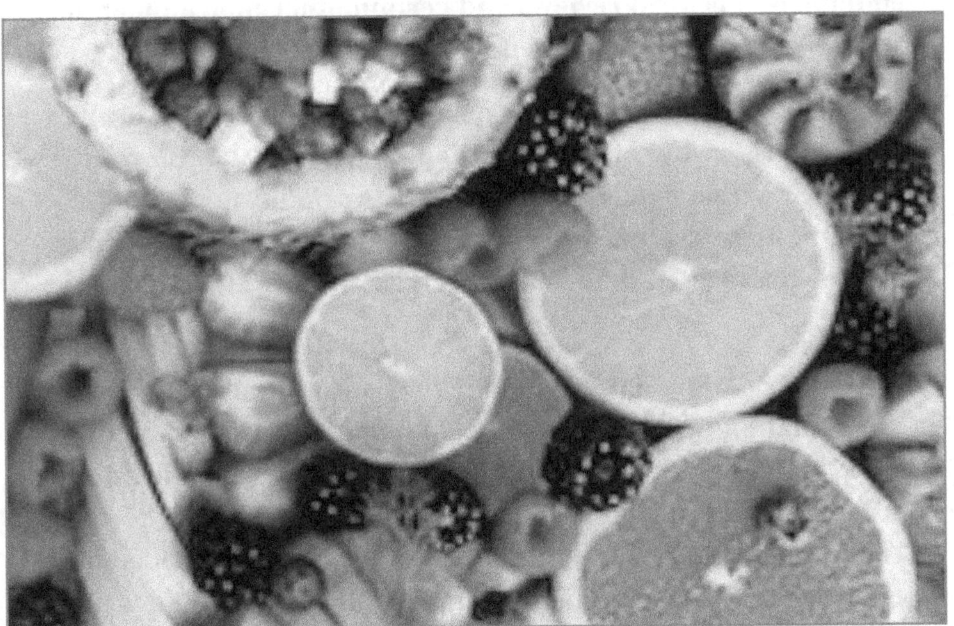

LAUREN WILLS

CONTENTS

INTRODUCTION

Welcome to "Brain-Boosting Recipes for Cognitive Wellness," a culinary journey designed to nourish not just your body, but also your mind. In the fast-paced world we live in, it's essential to prioritize our cognitive health. The food we eat has a profound impact on our mental well-being, influencing our focus, memory, mood, and overall cognitive function.

This cookbook is a testament to the idea that delicious and nutritious meals can go hand in hand. We've carefully curated a collection of 50 recipes that are not only satisfying to the palate but also packed with ingredients known to support cognitive health. Whether you're looking to sharpen your focus, enhance your memory, or simply maintain a clear and alert mind, these recipes are here to assist you on your journey.

Each recipe in this collection is crafted with ingredients rich in antioxidants, vitamins, minerals, and healthy fats—nutrients that have been scientifically linked to improved cognitive function. From vibrant salads and hearty soups to satisfying entrees and delightful desserts, there's a brain-boosting dish for every occasion.

We've included a variety of recipes to cater to different tastes and dietary preferences, ensuring that you can enjoy these nourishing meals regardless of your culinary background. Whether you're a seasoned chef or a novice in the kitchen, the step-by-step instructions make it easy for you to create these dishes with confidence.

In addition to tantalizing your taste buds and supporting your cognitive wellness, these recipes are designed to fit seamlessly into your busy life. We've included estimated prep times, nutritional values, and clear directions to help you make informed choices about the meals you prepare.

As you embark on this culinary adventure, we encourage you to savor each bite, be present in the moment, and appreciate the powerful connection between food and cognitive wellness. By choosing these brain-boosting recipes, you're making a conscious decision to invest in your mental vitality—one delicious meal at a time.

So, without further ado, let's dive into the world of "Brain-Boosting Recipes for Cognitive Wellness." May these dishes not only delight your taste buds but also enhance your cognitive potential, contributing to a life filled with clarity, focus, and vitality.

Here's to a healthier, happier, and more mentally vibrant you!

Bon appétit

BRAIN-BOOSTING RECIPES

Recipe 1: Blueberry Almond Overnight Oats

Prep Time: 10 minutes Yields: 2 servings

Ingredients:

- 1 cup rolled oats
- 1 cup almond milk
- 1/2 cup fresh blueberries
- 2 tablespoons honey
- 1/4 cup sliced almonds
- 1/2 teaspoon vanilla extract

Directions:

1. In a jar, combine rolled oats and almond milk.
2. Add blueberries, honey, sliced almonds, and vanilla extract.
3. Stir well, cover, and refrigerate overnight.
4. Serve chilled in the morning.

Nutritional Value (per serving):

- Calories: 350

- Protein: 8g

- Carbohydrates: 56g

- Fiber: 7g

- Fat: 12g

Recipe 2: Spinach and Mushroom Quiche

Prep Time: 30 minutes Yields: 6 servings

Ingredients:

- 1 pie crust

- 1 cup fresh spinach, chopped

- 1 cup mushrooms, sliced

- 1/2 cup grated Swiss cheese

- 4 large eggs

- 1 cup milk

- 1/2 teaspoon salt

- 1/4 teaspoon black pepper

Directions:

1. Preheat oven to 375°F (190°C).

2. Line the pie crust with spinach, mushrooms, and Swiss cheese.

3. In a bowl, whisk together eggs, milk, salt, and black pepper.

4. Pour the egg mixture over the spinach and mushrooms.

5. Bake for 25-30 minutes until set and golden.

6. Slice and serve.

Nutritional Value (per serving):

- Calories: 220

- Protein: 9g

- Carbohydrates: 16g

- Fiber: 1g

- Fat: 13g

Recipe 3: Salmon and Quinoa Salad

Prep Time: 20 minutes Yields: 4 servings

Ingredients:

- 2 cups cooked quinoa

- 2 grilled salmon fillets, flaked

- 1 cup cherry tomatoes, halved

- 1/2 cucumber, diced

- 1/4 cup red onion, finely chopped

- 1/4 cup fresh dill, chopped

- 1/4 cup lemon juice

- 2 tablespoons olive oil

- Salt and pepper to taste

Directions:

1. In a large bowl, combine quinoa, flaked salmon, cherry tomatoes, cucumber, red onion, and dill.

2. In a separate bowl, whisk together lemon juice, olive oil, salt, and pepper.

3. Drizzle the dressing over the salad and toss to combine.

4. Serve chilled.

Nutritional Value (per serving):

- Calories: 380

- Protein: 28g

- Carbohydrates: 30g

- Fiber: 4g

- Fat: 16g

Recipe 4: Avocado and Spinach Smoothie

Prep Time: 5 minutes Yields: 2 servings

Ingredients:

- 1 ripe avocado

- 2 cups fresh spinach

- 1 banana

- 1 cup almond milk

- 1 tablespoon honey

- 1/2 teaspoon cinnamon

Directions:

1. Blend avocado, spinach, banana, almond milk, honey, and cinnamon until smooth.

2. Pour into glasses and serve immediately.

Nutritional Value (per serving):

- Calories: 250

- Protein: 3g

- Carbohydrates: 31g

- Fiber: 8g

- Fat: 14g

Recipe 5: Broccoli and Cheddar Stuffed Sweet Potatoes

Prep Time: 45 minutes Yields: 4 servings

Ingredients:

- 4 medium sweet potatoes

- 2 cups steamed broccoli florets

- 1 cup shredded cheddar cheese

- 1/4 cup Greek yogurt

- 2 tablespoons chopped chives

- Salt and pepper to taste

Directions:

1. Preheat oven to 400°F (200°C).

2. Pierce sweet potatoes with a fork and bake for 40-45 minutes until tender.

3. Split the sweet potatoes and fluff the flesh.

4. Top with steamed broccoli, cheddar cheese, Greek yogurt, chives, salt, and pepper.

5. Serve hot.

Nutritional Value (per serving):

- Calories: 290

- Protein: 12g

- Carbohydrates: 39g

- Fiber: 6g

- Fat: 10g

Recipe 6: Berry Blast Chia Pudding

Prep Time: 15 minutes Yields: 2 servings

Ingredients:

- 1/4 cup chia seeds

- 1 cup almond milk

- 1/2 cup mixed berries (strawberries, blueberries, raspberries)

- 1 tablespoon maple syrup

- 1/2 teaspoon vanilla extract

Directions:

1. In a bowl, mix chia seeds, almond milk, maple syrup, and vanilla extract.

2. Refrigerate for at least 2 hours, or until the mixture thickens.

3. Layer chia pudding and mixed berries in serving glasses.

4. Repeat layers and top with extra berries if desired.

5. Serve chilled.

Nutritional Value (per serving):

- Calories: 220

- Protein: 5g

- Carbohydrates: 28g

- Fiber: 11g

- Fat: 9g

Recipe 7: Grilled Chicken and Vegetable Skewers

Prep Time: 25 minutes Yields: 4 servings

Ingredients:

- 1 pound boneless, skinless chicken breast, cut into chunks

- 1 red bell pepper, cut into chunks

- 1 yellow bell pepper, cut into chunks

- 1 red onion, cut into chunks

- 1 zucchini, sliced

- 1/4 cup olive oil

- 2 cloves garlic, minced

- 1 teaspoon dried oregano

- Salt and pepper to taste

Directions:

1. In a bowl, combine olive oil, minced garlic, oregano, salt, and pepper.

2. Thread chicken and vegetables onto skewers.

3. Brush skewers with the olive oil mixture.

4. Grill for 10-12 minutes, turning occasionally, until chicken is cooked through and vegetables are tender.

5. Serve hot.

Nutritional Value (per serving):

- Calories: 280

- Protein: 25g

- Carbohydrates: 10g

- Fiber: 2g

- Fat: 16g

Recipe 8: Quinoa and Black Bean Stuffed Peppers

Prep Time: 40 minutes Yields: 4 servings

Ingredients:

- 4 bell peppers, halved and seeds removed

- 1 cup cooked quinoa

- 1 cup black beans, drained and rinsed

- 1 cup corn kernels

- 1 cup diced tomatoes

- 1/2 cup shredded cheddar cheese

- 1 teaspoon chili powder

- 1/2 teaspoon cumin

- Salt and pepper to taste

Directions:

1. Preheat oven to 375°F (190°C).

2. In a bowl, combine cooked quinoa, black beans, corn, diced tomatoes, shredded cheddar cheese, chili powder, cumin, salt, and pepper.

3. Stuff the bell pepper halves with the quinoa mixture.

4. Place stuffed peppers in a baking dish, cover with foil, and bake for 25-30 minutes.

5. Remove foil and bake for an additional 5-10 minutes until peppers are tender and cheese is melted.

6. Serve hot.

Nutritional Value (per serving):

- Calories: 320

- Protein: 14g

- Carbohydrates: 54g

- Fiber: 11g

- Fat: 7g

Recipe 9: Wild Berry Parfait

Prep Time: 10 minutes Yields: 2 servings

Ingredients:

- 1 cup Greek yogurt

- 1/2 cup mixed wild berries (blackberries, raspberries)

- 1/4 cup granola

- 1 tablespoon honey

Directions:

1. In two serving glasses, layer Greek yogurt, mixed wild berries, and granola.

2. Drizzle honey over the top.

3. Repeat the layers if desired.

4. Serve chilled.

Nutritional Value (per serving):

- Calories: 250

- Protein: 14g

- Carbohydrates: 34g

- Fiber: 4g

- Fat: 6g

Recipe 10: Sweet Potato and Walnut Muffins

Prep Time: 15 minutes Baking Time: 25 minutes Yields: 12 muffins

Ingredients:

- 1 1/2 cups whole wheat flour

- 1 teaspoon baking powder

- 1/2 teaspoon baking soda

- 1/2 teaspoon cinnamon

- 1/4 teaspoon nutmeg

- 1/4 teaspoon salt

- 2 medium sweet potatoes, cooked and mashed

- 1/2 cup Greek yogurt

- 1/2 cup maple syrup

- 2 eggs

- 1/2 cup chopped walnuts

Directions:

1. Preheat oven to 350°F (175°C) and line a muffin tin with paper liners.

2. In a bowl, mix whole wheat flour, baking powder, baking soda, cinnamon, nutmeg, and salt.

3. In another bowl, combine mashed sweet potatoes, Greek yogurt, maple syrup, and eggs.

4. Gradually add the dry ingredients to the wet ingredients, mixing until just combined.

5. Fold in chopped walnuts.

6. Divide the batter evenly among the muffin cups.

7. Bake for 20-25 minutes, or until a toothpick inserted into the center comes out clean.

8. Allow muffins to cool before serving.

Nutritional Value (per muffin):

- Calories: 180

- Protein: 5g

- Carbohydrates: 28g

- Fiber: 3g

- Fat: 6g

Recipe 11: Coconut and Mango Chia Pudding

Prep Time: 10 minutes Yields: 2 servings

Ingredients:

- 1/4 cup chia seeds

- 1 cup coconut milk

- 1 ripe mango, diced

- 2 tablespoons shredded coconut

- 1 tablespoon agave syrup

- 1/2 teaspoon vanilla extract

Directions:

1. In a bowl, mix chia seeds, coconut milk, agave syrup, and vanilla extract.

2. Refrigerate for at least 2 hours or until thickened.

3. Layer chia pudding with diced mango and top with shredded coconut.

4. Serve chilled.

Nutritional Value (per serving):

- Calories: 280

- Protein: 4g

- Carbohydrates: 35g

- Fiber: 11g

- Fat: 15g

Recipe 12: Roasted Vegetable and Quinoa Bowl

Prep Time: 30 minutes Yields: 4 servings

Ingredients:

- 2 cups cooked quinoa

- 1 sweet potato, diced

- 1 red bell pepper, sliced

- 1 zucchini, sliced

- 1 red onion, sliced

- 2 tablespoons olive oil

- 1 teaspoon smoked paprika

- Salt and pepper to taste

- 1/4 cup feta cheese, crumbled

- 1/4 cup fresh basil, chopped

Directions:

1. Preheat oven to 425°F (220°C).

2. Toss sweet potato, red bell pepper, zucchini, and red onion with olive oil, smoked paprika, salt, and pepper.

3. Spread vegetables on a baking sheet and roast for 20-25 minutes, stirring occasionally, until tender and slightly crispy.

4. Divide quinoa among bowls, top with roasted vegetables, feta cheese, and fresh basil.

5. Serve warm.

Nutritional Value (per serving):

- Calories: 320

- Protein: 8g

- Carbohydrates: 46g

- Fiber: 7g

- Fat: 13g

Recipe 13: Almond Butter and Banana Smoothie

Prep Time: 5 minutes Yields: 2 servings

Ingredients:

- 2 ripe bananas

- 2 tablespoons almond butter

- 1 cup almond milk

- 1/2 cup Greek yogurt

- 1 tablespoon honey

- 1/2 teaspoon cinnamon

Directions:

1. Blend bananas, almond butter, almond milk, Greek yogurt, honey, and cinnamon until smooth.

2. Pour into glasses and serve immediately.

Nutritional Value (per serving):

- Calories: 290

- Protein: 7g

- Carbohydrates: 40g

- Fiber: 6g

- Fat: 12g

Recipe 14: Lemon Garlic Shrimp and Asparagus

Prep Time: 20 minutes Yields: 4 servings

Ingredients:

- 1 pound large shrimp, peeled and deveined

- 1 bunch asparagus, trimmed

- 2 tablespoons olive oil

- 2 cloves garlic, minced

- Zest and juice of 1 lemon

- Salt and pepper to taste

- Fresh parsley for garnish

Directions:

1. In a bowl, toss shrimp and asparagus with olive oil, minced garlic, lemon zest, lemon juice, salt, and pepper.

2. Heat a skillet over medium-high heat.

3. Add shrimp and asparagus to the skillet and cook for 3-4 minutes per side until shrimp are pink and asparagus is tender.

4. Garnish with fresh parsley and serve hot.

Nutritional Value (per serving):

- Calories: 210

- Protein: 24g

- Carbohydrates: 6g

- Fiber: 2g

- Fat: 10g

Recipe 15: Berry and Spinach Salad

Prep Time: 15 minutes Yields: 2 servings

Ingredients:

- 2 cups baby spinach

- 1/2 cup strawberries, sliced

- 1/2 cup blueberries

- 1/4 cup goat cheese, crumbled

- 1/4 cup chopped pecans

- Balsamic vinaigrette dressing

Directions:

1. In a bowl, combine baby spinach, strawberries, blueberries, goat cheese, and chopped pecans.

2. Drizzle with balsamic vinaigrette dressing and toss to coat.

3. Serve immediately.

Nutritional Value (per serving):

- Calories: 260

- Protein: 6g

- Carbohydrates: 17g

- Fiber: 4g

- Fat: 20g

Recipe 16: Mediterranean Quinoa Salad

Prep Time: 15 minutes Yields: 4 servings

Ingredients:

- 2 cups cooked quinoa

- 1 cup cucumber, diced

- 1 cup cherry tomatoes, halved

- 1/2 cup Kalamata olives, pitted and sliced

- 1/2 cup crumbled feta cheese

- 1/4 cup red onion, finely chopped

- 2 tablespoons olive oil

- 2 tablespoons lemon juice

- 1 teaspoon dried oregano

- Salt and pepper to taste

Directions:

1. In a bowl, combine cooked quinoa, cucumber, cherry tomatoes, Kalamata olives, feta cheese, and red onion.

2. In a separate bowl, whisk together olive oil, lemon juice, dried oregano, salt, and pepper.

3. Drizzle the dressing over the salad and toss to combine.

4. Serve chilled.

Nutritional Value (per serving):

- Calories: 330

- Protein: 9g

- Carbohydrates: 38g

- Fiber: 5g

- Fat: 17g

Recipe 17: Walnut and Blueberry Pancakes

Prep Time: 20 minutes Cook Time: 15 minutes Yields: 4 servings

Ingredients:

- 1 cup whole wheat flour

- 1/2 cup chopped walnuts

- 1 tablespoon baking powder

- 1/2 teaspoon cinnamon

- 1/4 teaspoon salt

- 1 cup almond milk

- 1 egg

- 2 tablespoons honey

- 1 cup blueberries (fresh or frozen)

Directions:

1. In a bowl, mix whole wheat flour, chopped walnuts, baking powder, cinnamon, and salt.

2. In another bowl, whisk together almond milk, egg, and honey.

3. Pour the wet ingredients into the dry ingredients and stir until just combined.

4. Gently fold in blueberries.

5. Heat a non-stick skillet over medium heat and lightly grease with cooking spray.

6. Pour 1/4 cup of batter for each pancake onto the skillet.

7. Cook for 2-3 minutes per side until golden brown.

8. Serve with additional blueberries and a drizzle of honey.

Nutritional Value (per serving):

- Calories: 320

- Protein: 9g

- Carbohydrates: 48g

- Fiber: 6g

- Fat: 11g

Recipe 18: Mediterranean Chickpea Salad

Prep Time: 15 minutes Yields: 4 servings

Ingredients:

- 2 cans (15 ounces each) chickpeas, drained and rinsed

- 1 cucumber, diced

- 1 cup cherry tomatoes, halved

- 1/2 cup red bell pepper, diced

- 1/4 cup red onion, finely chopped

- 1/4 cup fresh parsley, chopped

- 1/4 cup feta cheese, crumbled

- 2 tablespoons olive oil

- 2 tablespoons lemon juice

- 1 teaspoon dried oregano

- Salt and pepper to taste

Directions:

1. In a bowl, combine chickpeas, cucumber, cherry tomatoes, red bell pepper, red onion, fresh parsley, and feta cheese.

2. In a separate bowl, whisk together olive oil, lemon juice, dried oregano, salt, and pepper.

3. Drizzle the dressing over the salad and toss to combine.

4. Serve chilled.

Nutritional Value (per serving):

- Calories: 320

- Protein: 12g

- Carbohydrates: 44g

- Fiber: 11g

- Fat: 13g

Recipe 19: Tomato and Basil Bruschetta

Prep Time: 15 minutes Yields: 4 servings

Ingredients:

- 4 slices whole wheat baguette

- 2 cups diced tomatoes

- 1/4 cup fresh basil leaves, chopped

- 2 cloves garlic, minced

- 2 tablespoons extra virgin olive oil

- Salt and pepper to taste

- Balsamic glaze for drizzling (optional)

Directions:

1. Preheat oven to 350°F (175°C).

2. Place baguette slices on a baking sheet and toast for 5-7 minutes until lightly crisp.

3. In a bowl, combine diced tomatoes, fresh basil, minced garlic, extra virgin olive oil, salt, and pepper.

4. Spoon the tomato mixture onto the toasted baguette slices.

5. Drizzle with balsamic glaze if desired.

6. Serve immediately.

Nutritional Value (per serving):

- Calories: 160

- Protein: 3g

- Carbohydrates: 19g

- Fiber: 2g

- Fat: 8g

Recipe 20: Green Tea and Berry Smoothie

Prep Time: 10 minutes Yields: 2 servings

Ingredients:

- 1 cup brewed green tea, cooled

- 1 cup mixed berries (strawberries, blueberries, raspberries)

- 1 banana

- 1/2 cup Greek yogurt

- 1 tablespoon honey

- 1/2 teaspoon matcha powder (optional)

Directions:

1. Blend green tea, mixed berries, banana, Greek yogurt, honey, and matcha powder (if using) until smooth.

2. Pour into glasses and serve immediately.

Nutritional Value (per serving):

- Calories: 180

- Protein: 7g

- Carbohydrates: 38g

- Fiber: 5g

- Fat: 1g

Recipe 21: Kale and Pomegranate Salad

Prep Time: 15 minutes Yields: 4 servings

Ingredients:

- 4 cups kale leaves, chopped

- 1/2 cup pomegranate seeds

- 1/4 cup feta cheese, crumbled

- 1/4 cup chopped walnuts

- 2 tablespoons olive oil

- 2 tablespoons lemon juice

- 1 teaspoon honey

- Salt and pepper to taste

Directions:

1. In a bowl, massage kale leaves with olive oil and lemon juice for a few minutes to soften.

2. Add pomegranate seeds, crumbled feta cheese, chopped walnuts, honey, salt, and pepper.

3. Toss to combine and serve immediately.

Nutritional Value (per serving):

- Calories: 240

- Protein: 7g

- Carbohydrates: 18g

- Fiber: 4g

- Fat: 17g

Recipe 22: Mediterranean Stuffed Bell Peppers

Prep Time: 30 minutes Cook Time: 25 minutes Yields: 4 servings

Ingredients:

- 4 large bell peppers, any color

- 1 cup cooked quinoa

- 1 can (15 ounces) chickpeas, drained and rinsed

- 1 cup diced tomatoes

- 1/2 cup Kalamata olives, pitted and sliced

- 1/4 cup crumbled feta cheese

- 1/4 cup fresh parsley, chopped

- 2 tablespoons olive oil

- 1 teaspoon dried oregano

- Salt and pepper to taste

Directions:

1. Preheat oven to 375°F (190°C).

2. Cut the tops off the bell peppers and remove the seeds.

3. In a bowl, combine cooked quinoa, chickpeas, diced tomatoes, Kalamata olives, feta cheese, fresh parsley, olive oil, dried oregano, salt, and pepper.

4. Stuff the bell peppers with the quinoa mixture.

5. Place stuffed peppers in a baking dish, cover with foil, and bake for 20-25 minutes.

6. Remove foil and bake for an additional 5 minutes until peppers are tender and filling is heated through.

7. Serve hot.

Nutritional Value (per serving):

- Calories: 380

- Protein: 13g

- Carbohydrates: 54g

- Fiber: 11g

- Fat: 14g

Recipe 23: Apple and Cinnamon Oatmeal

Prep Time: 10 minutes Cook Time: 10 minutes Yields: 2 servings

Ingredients:

- 1 cup rolled oats

- 2 cups water

- 1 apple, peeled, cored, and diced

- 1/2 teaspoon ground cinnamon

- 1/4 teaspoon nutmeg

- 2 tablespoons maple syrup

- 1/4 cup chopped walnuts

- 1/4 cup raisins

Directions:

1. In a saucepan, combine rolled oats, water, diced apple, ground cinnamon, and nutmeg.

2. Bring to a boil, then reduce heat and simmer for 5-7 minutes, stirring occasionally, until oats are cooked and apple is tender.

3. Stir in maple syrup, chopped walnuts, and raisins.

4. Serve hot.

Nutritional Value (per serving):

- Calories: 330

- Protein: 8g

- Carbohydrates: 63g

- Fiber: 7g

- Fat: 7g

Recipe 24: Roasted Beet and Goat Cheese Salad

Prep Time: 20 minutes Cook Time: 45 minutes Yields: 4 servings

Ingredients:

- 4 medium beets, peeled and diced

- 2 tablespoons olive oil

- Salt and pepper to taste

- 4 cups mixed greens

- 1/2 cup crumbled goat cheese

- 1/4 cup chopped pecans

- Balsamic vinaigrette dressing

Directions:

1. Preheat oven to 400°F (200°C).

2. Toss diced beets with olive oil, salt, and pepper.

3. Spread beets on a baking sheet and roast for 40-45 minutes until tender.

4. In a bowl, assemble mixed greens, roasted beets, crumbled goat cheese, and chopped pecans.

5. Drizzle with balsamic vinaigrette dressing.

6. Serve immediately.

Nutritional Value (per serving):

- Calories: 250

- Protein: 7g

- Carbohydrates: 14g

- Fiber: 4g

- Fat: 19g

Recipe 25: Berry and Avocado Spinach Salad

Prep Time: 15 minutes Yields: 2 servings

Ingredients:

- 4 cups baby spinach

- 1/2 cup mixed berries (strawberries, blueberries, raspberries)

- 1/2 avocado, diced

- 1/4 cup red onion, thinly sliced

- 1/4 cup crumbled feta cheese

- 2 tablespoons balsamic vinaigrette dressing

Directions:

1. In a bowl, combine baby spinach, mixed berries, diced avocado, thinly sliced red onion, and crumbled feta cheese.

2. Drizzle with balsamic vinaigrette dressing and toss to coat.

3. Serve immediately.

Nutritional Value (per serving):

- Calories: 280

- Protein: 7g

- Carbohydrates: 20g

- Fiber: 6g

- Fat: 20g

Recipe 26: Quinoa and Blackberry Salad

Prep Time: 15 minutes Yields: 4 servings

Ingredients:

- 2 cups cooked quinoa

- 1 cup blackberries

- 1/2 cup cucumber, diced

- 1/4 cup red onion, finely chopped

- 1/4 cup fresh mint leaves, chopped

- 2 tablespoons olive oil

- 2 tablespoons lemon juice

- Salt and pepper to taste

Directions:

1. In a bowl, combine cooked quinoa, blackberries, diced cucumber, finely chopped red onion, and fresh mint leaves.

2. In a separate bowl, whisk together olive oil, lemon juice, salt, and pepper.

3. Drizzle the dressing over the salad and toss to combine.

4. Serve chilled.

Nutritional Value (per serving):

- Calories: 280

- Protein: 5g

- Carbohydrates: 42g

- Fiber: 8g

- Fat: 10g

Recipe 27: Avocado and Egg Breakfast Sandwich

Prep Time: 15 minutes Yields: 2 servings

Ingredients:

- 4 slices whole grain bread

- 1 ripe avocado, mashed

- 4 boiled eggs, sliced

- 1/2 cup baby spinach leaves

- Salt and pepper to taste

- Hot sauce (optional)

Directions:

1. Toast the whole grain bread slices.

2. Spread mashed avocado on two slices.

3. Layer sliced boiled eggs and baby spinach leaves on the avocado.

4. Season with salt, pepper, and hot sauce if desired.

5. Top with the remaining bread slices to make sandwiches.

6. Serve immediately.

Nutritional Value (per serving):

- Calories: 370

- Protein: 18g

- Carbohydrates: 32g

- Fiber: 11g

- Fat: 21g

Recipe 28: Quinoa and Vegetable Stir-Fry

Prep Time: 20 minutes Cook Time: 15 minutes Yields: 4 servings

Ingredients:

- 1 cup cooked quinoa

- 1 cup broccoli florets

- 1 cup bell peppers, sliced

- 1 cup snap peas

- 1/2 cup carrots, thinly sliced

- 1/4 cup low-sodium soy sauce

- 2 tablespoons olive oil

- 1 tablespoon honey

- 2 cloves garlic, minced

- 1 teaspoon ginger, minced

- Sesame seeds for garnish

Directions:

1. In a wok or large skillet, heat olive oil over high heat.

2. Add minced garlic and ginger, and stir-fry for 30 seconds.

3. Add broccoli florets, bell peppers, snap peas, and sliced carrots.

4. Stir-fry for 5-7 minutes until vegetables are tender-crisp.

5. In a small bowl, whisk together low-sodium soy sauce, honey, and a splash of water.

6. Add cooked quinoa to the wok and pour the soy sauce mixture over the quinoa and vegetables.

7. Toss to combine and cook for an additional 2-3 minutes.

8. Garnish with sesame seeds and serve hot.

Nutritional Value (per serving):

- Calories: 290

- Protein: 7g

- Carbohydrates: 44g

- Fiber: 6g

- Fat: 9g

Recipe 29: Tomato and Basil Frittata

Prep Time: 15 minutes Cook Time: 20 minutes Yields: 4 servings

Ingredients:

- 6 large eggs

- 1 cup cherry tomatoes, halved

- 1/4 cup fresh basil leaves, chopped

- 1/4 cup grated Parmesan cheese

- Salt and pepper to taste

- 1 tablespoon olive oil

Directions:

1. Preheat the broiler.

2. In a bowl, whisk eggs, cherry tomatoes, fresh basil, grated Parmesan cheese, salt, and pepper.

3. Heat olive oil in an ovenproof skillet over medium heat.

4. Pour the egg mixture into the skillet and cook for 5-7 minutes until the edges are set.

5. Transfer the skillet to the broiler and broil for 3-5 minutes until the top is golden and the center is set.

6. Slice into wedges and serve hot or at room temperature.

Nutritional Value (per serving):

- Calories: 200

- Protein: 13g

- Carbohydrates: 4g

- Fiber: 1g

- Fat: 15g

Recipe 30: Sweet Potato and Chickpea Curry

Prep Time: 15 minutes Cook Time: 25 minutes Yields: 4 servings

Ingredients:

- 2 sweet potatoes, peeled and diced

- 1 can (15 ounces) chickpeas, drained and rinsed

- 1 onion, finely chopped

- 2 cloves garlic, minced

- 1 tablespoon curry powder

- 1/2 teaspoon cumin

- 1/2 teaspoon turmeric

- 1/2 teaspoon paprika

- 1 can (14 ounces) diced tomatoes

- 1 can (14 ounces) coconut milk

- Salt and pepper to taste

- Fresh cilantro for garnish

Directions:

1. In a large pot, sauté onion and garlic in olive oil over medium heat until translucent.

2. Add curry powder, cumin, turmeric, and paprika, and cook for 1-2 minutes until fragrant.

3. Stir in diced sweet potatoes, chickpeas, diced tomatoes, and coconut milk.

4. Simmer for 20-25 minutes until sweet potatoes are tender.

5. Season with salt and pepper.

6. Serve hot, garnished with fresh cilantro.

Nutritional Value (per serving):

- Calories: 350

- Protein: 9g

- Carbohydrates: 46g

- Fiber: 10g

- Fat: 16g

Recipe 31: Spinach and Mushroom Stuffed Chicken

Prep Time: 20 minutes Cook Time: 25 minutes Yields: 4 servings

Ingredients:

- 4 boneless, skinless chicken breasts

- 2 cups fresh spinach leaves

- 1 cup mushrooms, sliced

- 1/2 cup shredded mozzarella cheese

- 2 cloves garlic, minced

- 1 tablespoon olive oil

- Salt and pepper to taste

- Toothpicks for securing

Directions:

1. Preheat oven to 375°F (190°C).

2. In a skillet, heat olive oil over medium heat. Add minced garlic and sliced mushrooms, sauté for 3-4 minutes until mushrooms are tender.

3. Add fresh spinach leaves to the skillet and cook for another 2 minutes until wilted. Season with salt and pepper.

4. Butterfly each chicken breast by slicing horizontally, then stuff with the spinach and mushroom mixture and a sprinkle of mozzarella cheese.

5. Secure with toothpicks.

6. Heat a large ovenproof skillet over medium-high heat, and sear the stuffed chicken breasts for 2-3 minutes per side until browned.

7. Transfer the skillet to the preheated oven and bake for 15-20 minutes until chicken is cooked through.

8. Remove toothpicks before serving.

Nutritional Value (per serving):

- Calories: 260

- Protein: 34g

- Carbohydrates: 4g

- Fiber: 1g

- Fat: 11g

Recipe 32: Lemon Garlic Roasted Salmon

Prep Time: 10 minutes Cook Time: 15 minutes Yields: 4 servings

Ingredients:

- 4 salmon fillets

- 2 lemons, sliced

- 4 cloves garlic, minced

- 2 tablespoons olive oil

- 1 teaspoon dried oregano

- Salt and pepper to taste

- Fresh parsley for garnish

Directions:

1. Preheat oven to 400°F (200°C).

2. In a bowl, mix minced garlic, olive oil, dried oregano, salt, and pepper.

3. Place salmon fillets on a baking sheet lined with parchment paper.

4. Brush the garlic and herb mixture over the salmon.

5. Arrange lemon slices on top.

6. Bake for 12-15 minutes until salmon flakes easily with a fork.

7. Garnish with fresh parsley before serving.

Nutritional Value (per serving):

- Calories: 290

- Protein: 34g

- Carbohydrates: 5g

- Fiber: 2g

- Fat: 15g

Recipe 33: Berry and Almond Butter Overnight Oats

Prep Time: 10 minutes Chill Time: Overnight Yields: 2 servings

Ingredients:

- 1 cup rolled oats

- 1 1/2 cups almond milk

- 2 tablespoons almond butter

- 1/2 cup mixed berries (strawberries, blueberries, raspberries)

- 1 tablespoon honey

- 1/4 cup sliced almonds

Directions:

1. In a jar or container, combine rolled oats, almond milk, almond butter, mixed berries, and honey.

2. Stir well, cover, and refrigerate overnight.

3. In the morning, give the oats a good stir, and top with sliced almonds before serving.

Nutritional Value (per serving):

- Calories: 340

- Protein: 9g

- Carbohydrates: 44g

- Fiber: 8g

- Fat: 16g

Recipe 34: Turkey and Spinach Stuffed Portobello Mushrooms

Prep Time: 20 minutes Cook Time: 25 minutes Yields: 4 servings

Ingredients:

- 4 large Portobello mushrooms, stems removed

- 1 pound ground turkey

- 2 cups fresh spinach leaves

- 1/2 cup diced tomatoes

- 1/4 cup shredded mozzarella cheese

- 2 cloves garlic, minced

- 2 tablespoons olive oil

- Salt and pepper to taste

Directions:

1. Preheat oven to 375°F (190°C).

2. Brush Portobello mushroom caps with olive oil and season with salt and pepper.

3. Place mushrooms on a baking sheet and bake for 10 minutes.

4. In a skillet, heat olive oil over medium heat. Add minced garlic and ground turkey, cook until browned and cooked through.

5. Add fresh spinach leaves and diced tomatoes to the skillet, and cook for another 2 minutes until spinach wilts. Season with salt and pepper.

6. Remove the mushroom caps from the oven and stuff with the turkey, spinach, and tomato mixture.

7. Top each stuffed mushroom with shredded mozzarella cheese.

8. Bake for an additional 15 minutes until cheese is melted and mushrooms are tender.

9. Serve hot.

Nutritional Value (per serving):

- Calories: 320

- Protein: 31g

- Carbohydrates: 7g

- Fiber: 2g

- Fat: 18g

Recipe 35: Blueberry and Banana Muffins

Prep Time: 15 minutes Baking Time: 25 minutes Yields: 12 muffins

Ingredients:

- 1 1/2 cups whole wheat flour

- 1/2 cup rolled oats

- 1/2 cup blueberries (fresh or frozen)

- 2 ripe bananas, mashed

- 1/2 cup Greek yogurt

- 1/4 cup honey

- 1/4 cup unsweetened applesauce

- 2 eggs

- 1 teaspoon baking powder

- 1/2 teaspoon baking soda

- 1/2 teaspoon cinnamon

- 1/4 teaspoon salt

Directions:

1. Preheat oven to 350°F (175°C) and line a muffin tin with paper liners.

2. In a bowl, mix whole wheat flour, rolled oats, baking powder, baking soda, cinnamon, and salt.

3. In another bowl, combine mashed bananas, Greek yogurt, honey, unsweetened applesauce, and eggs.

4. Gradually add the dry ingredients to the wet ingredients, mixing until just combined.

5. Gently fold in blueberries.

6. Divide the batter evenly among the muffin cups.

7. Bake for 20-25 minutes, or until a toothpick inserted into the center comes out clean.

8. Allow muffins to cool before serving.

Nutritional Value (per muffin):

- Calories: 160

- Protein: 4g

- Carbohydrates: 30g

- Fiber: 4g

- Fat: 3g

Recipe 36: Lentil and Vegetable Soup

Prep Time: 15 minutes Cook Time: 30 minutes Yields: 4 servings

Ingredients:

- 1 cup dried green lentils

- 1 onion, finely chopped

- 2 carrots, diced

- 2 celery stalks, diced

- 2 cloves garlic, minced

- 6 cups vegetable broth

- 1 can (14 ounces) diced tomatoes

- 1 teaspoon dried thyme

- 1/2 teaspoon cumin

- Salt and pepper to taste

- Fresh parsley for garnish

Directions:

1. Rinse lentils under cold water and set aside.

2. In a large pot, sauté chopped onion, diced carrots, and diced celery in olive oil over medium heat until softened.

3. Add minced garlic and cook for another minute until fragrant.

4. Add lentils, vegetable broth, diced tomatoes, dried thyme, cumin, salt, and pepper to the pot.

5. Bring to a boil, then reduce heat to a simmer and cook for 25-30 minutes until lentils are tender.

6. Garnish with fresh parsley before serving.

Nutritional Value (per serving):

- Calories: 280

- Protein: 16g

- Carbohydrates: 50g

- Fiber: 18g

- Fat: 1g

Recipe 37: Caprese Stuffed Avocado

Prep Time: 10 minutes Yields: 2 servings

Ingredients:

- 2 ripe avocados

- 1 cup cherry tomatoes, halved

- 1/2 cup fresh mozzarella balls

- 1/4 cup fresh basil leaves, torn

- Balsamic glaze for drizzling

- Salt and pepper to taste

Directions:

1. Cut avocados in half and remove the pits.

2. Scoop out some of the flesh from each avocado half to create a larger cavity.

3. In a bowl, combine cherry tomatoes, fresh mozzarella balls, and torn basil leaves.

4. Season with salt and pepper.

5. Fill each avocado half with the tomato and mozzarella mixture.

6. Drizzle with balsamic glaze.

7. Serve immediately.

Nutritional Value (per serving):

- Calories: 280

- Protein: 10g

- Carbohydrates: 12g

- Fiber: 7g

- Fat: 23g

Recipe 38: Garlic Herb Roasted Vegetables

Prep Time: 15 minutes Cook Time: 30 minutes Yields: 4 servings

Ingredients:

- 2 cups baby potatoes, halved

- 2 cups baby carrots

- 2 cups green beans, trimmed

- 1 red bell pepper, sliced

- 1 yellow bell pepper, sliced

- 3 cloves garlic, minced

- 2 tablespoons olive oil

- 1 teaspoon dried rosemary

- 1 teaspoon dried thyme

- Salt and pepper to taste

- Fresh parsley for garnish

Directions:

1. Preheat oven to 425°F (220°C).

2. In a large bowl, combine baby potatoes, baby carrots, green beans, sliced red bell pepper, sliced yellow bell pepper, minced garlic, olive oil, dried rosemary, dried thyme, salt, and pepper.

3. Toss until vegetables are coated with the olive oil and seasoning.

4. Spread the vegetables on a baking sheet in a single layer.

5. Roast for 25-30 minutes, stirring once halfway through, until vegetables are tender and slightly crispy.

6. Garnish with fresh parsley before serving.

Nutritional Value (per serving):

- Calories: 190

- Protein: 3g

- Carbohydrates: 26g

- Fiber: 6g

- Fat: 9g

Recipe 39: Peanut Butter and Banana Smoothie Bowl

Prep Time: 10 minutes Yields: 2 servings

Ingredients:

- 2 ripe bananas

- 1/4 cup peanut butter

- 1 cup Greek yogurt

- 1/2 cup almond milk

- 2 tablespoons honey

- 1/4 cup granola

- 1/4 cup mixed berries (strawberries, blueberries, raspberries)

Directions:

1. In a blender, combine ripe bananas, peanut butter, Greek yogurt, almond milk, and honey.

2. Blend until smooth and creamy.

3. Pour the smoothie into bowls.

4. Top with granola and mixed berries.

5. Serve immediately.

Nutritional Value (per serving):

- Calories: 410

- Protein: 15g

- Carbohydrates: 47g

- Fiber: 6g

- Fat: 19g

Recipe 40: Roasted Red Pepper and Chickpea Hummus

Prep Time: 10 minutes Yields: 2 cups

Ingredients:

- 1 can (15 ounces) chickpeas, drained and rinsed

- 2 roasted red peppers, peeled and seeded

- 2 cloves garlic

- 2 tablespoons tahini

- 2 tablespoons lemon juice

- 1/4 cup olive oil

- 1/2 teaspoon cumin

- Salt and pepper to taste

- Paprika for garnish

- Fresh parsley for garnish

Directions:

1. In a food processor, combine chickpeas, roasted red peppers, garlic, tahini, lemon juice, olive oil, cumin, salt, and pepper.

2. Process until smooth and creamy.

3. Transfer to a serving bowl.

4. Garnish with paprika and fresh parsley.

5. Serve with pita bread, carrot sticks, or cucumber slices.

Nutritional Value (per 2-tablespoon serving):

- Calories: 70

- Protein: 2g

- Carbohydrates: 5g

- Fiber: 1g

- Fat: 5g

Recipe 41: Tuna and White Bean Salad

Prep Time: 15 minutes Yields: 4 servings

Ingredients:

- 2 cans (5 ounces each) tuna, drained

- 1 can (15 ounces) cannellini beans, drained and rinsed

- 1/2 cup cherry tomatoes, halved

- 1/4 cup red onion, finely chopped

- 1/4 cup fresh basil leaves, chopped

- 2 tablespoons olive oil

- 2 tablespoons red wine vinegar

- Salt and pepper to taste

- Lemon wedges for garnish

Directions:

1. In a bowl, combine drained tuna, cannellini beans, cherry tomatoes, red onion, and fresh basil.

2. In a small bowl, whisk together olive oil and red wine vinegar.

3. Pour the dressing over the salad and toss to combine.

4. Season with salt and pepper.

5. Garnish with lemon wedges before serving.

Nutritional Value (per serving):

- Calories: 280

- Protein: 27g

- Carbohydrates: 21g

- Fiber: 6g

- Fat: 10g

Recipe 42: Mango and Quinoa Salad

Prep Time: 15 minutes Yields: 4 servings

Ingredients:

- 1 cup cooked quinoa

- 2 ripe mangoes, diced

- 1 red bell pepper, diced

- 1/4 cup red onion, finely chopped

- 1/4 cup fresh cilantro, chopped

- 2 tablespoons lime juice

- 2 tablespoons olive oil

- Salt and pepper to taste

Directions:

1. In a bowl, combine cooked quinoa, diced mangoes, diced red bell pepper, finely chopped red onion, and chopped fresh cilantro.

2. In a small bowl, whisk together lime juice, olive oil, salt, and pepper.

Brain-Boosting Recipes Cookbook for Cognitive Wellness

3. Drizzle the dressing over the salad and toss to combine.

4. Serve chilled.

Nutritional Value (per serving):

- Calories: 250

- Protein: 4g

- Carbohydrates: 42g

- Fiber: 5g

- Fat: 9g

Recipe 43: Turkey and Vegetable Stir-Fry

Prep Time: 20 minutes Cook Time: 15 minutes Yields: 4 servings

Ingredients:

- 1 pound lean ground turkey

- 2 cups broccoli florets

- 1 cup bell peppers, sliced

- 1 cup snap peas

- 1/2 cup carrots, thinly sliced

- 1/4 cup low-sodium soy sauce

- 2 tablespoons olive oil

- 1 tablespoon honey

- 2 cloves garlic, minced

- 1 teaspoon ginger, minced

- Sesame seeds for garnish

Directions:

1. In a large skillet, heat olive oil over high heat.

2. Add minced garlic and ginger, and stir-fry for 30 seconds.

3. Add ground turkey and cook until browned and cooked through.

4. Add broccoli florets, bell peppers, snap peas, and sliced carrots.

5. Stir-fry for 5-7 minutes until vegetables are tender-crisp.

6. In a small bowl, whisk together low-sodium soy sauce, honey, and a splash of water.

7. Pour the sauce over the turkey and vegetables.

8. Toss to combine and cook for an additional 2-3
   minutes.

9. Garnish with sesame seeds and serve hot.

Nutritional Value (per serving):

- Calories: 290

- Protein: 23g

- Carbohydrates: 18g

- Fiber: 4g

- Fat: 15g

Recipe 44: Cucumber and Dill Greek Yogurt Dip
Prep Time: 10 minutes Yields: 2 cups

Ingredients:

- 2 cups Greek yogurt

- 1 cucumber, grated

- 2 cloves garlic, minced

- 2 tablespoons fresh dill, chopped

- 1 tablespoon lemon juice

- Salt and pepper to taste

- Fresh cucumber slices and cherry tomatoes for dipping

Directions:

1. In a bowl, combine Greek yogurt, grated cucumber, minced garlic, chopped fresh dill, lemon juice, salt, and pepper.

2. Mix until well combined.

3. Refrigerate for at least 30 minutes to allow the flavors to meld.

4. Serve with cucumber slices and cherry tomatoes for dipping.

Nutritional Value (per 2-tablespoon serving):

- Calories: 25

- Protein: 2g

- Carbohydrates: 3g

- Fiber: 0g

- Fat: 0g

Recipe 45: Asian-Inspired Quinoa Salad

Prep Time: 15 minutes Yields: 4 servings

Ingredients:

- 2 cups cooked quinoa

- 1 cup shredded cabbage

- 1/2 cup shredded carrots

- 1/2 cup edamame beans, shelled

- 1/4 cup chopped scallions

- 2 tablespoons sesame oil

- 2 tablespoons low-sodium soy sauce

- 1 tablespoon rice vinegar

- 1 teaspoon honey

- 1/2 teaspoon ginger, minced

- Sesame seeds for garnish

Directions:

1. In a bowl, combine cooked quinoa, shredded cabbage, shredded carrots, edamame beans, and chopped scallions.

2. In a small bowl, whisk together sesame oil, low-sodium soy sauce, rice vinegar, honey, and minced ginger.

3. Pour the dressing over the salad and toss to combine.

4. Garnish with sesame seeds before serving.

Nutritional Value (per serving):

- Calories: 260

- Protein: 9g

- Carbohydrates: 33g

- Fiber: 5g

- Fat: 11g

Recipe 46: Broccoli and Cheddar Stuffed Sweet Potatoes

Prep Time: 15 minutes Cook Time: 45 minutes Yields: 4 servings

Ingredients:

- 4 medium sweet potatoes

- 2 cups broccoli florets, steamed

- 1 cup shredded cheddar cheese

- 1/4 cup Greek yogurt

- Salt and pepper to taste

- Fresh chives for garnish

Directions:

1. Preheat oven to 400°F (200°C).

2. Scrub sweet potatoes, pierce with a fork, and bake for 40-45 minutes until tender.

3. Cut a slit in the top of each sweet potato and fluff the insides with a fork.

4. Top with steamed broccoli florets, shredded cheddar cheese, and a dollop of Greek yogurt.

5. Season with salt and pepper.

6. Garnish with fresh chives before serving.

Nutritional Value (per serving):

- Calories: 290

- Protein: 13g

- Carbohydrates: 45g

- Fiber: 7g

- Fat: 8g

Recipe 47: Spinach and Feta Stuffed Chicken Breast

Prep Time: 20 minutes Cook Time: 25 minutes Yields: 4 servings

Ingredients:

- 4 boneless, skinless chicken breasts

- 2 cups fresh spinach leaves

- 1/2 cup crumbled feta cheese

- 2 cloves garlic, minced

- 2 tablespoons olive oil

- Salt and pepper to taste

- Toothpicks for securing

Directions:

1. Preheat oven to 375°F (190°C).

2. In a skillet, heat olive oil over medium heat. Add minced garlic and fresh spinach, sauté for 2-3 minutes until spinach wilts. Season with salt and pepper.

3. Butterfly each chicken breast by slicing horizontally, then stuff with the spinach and feta mixture.

4. Secure with toothpicks.

5. Heat a large ovenproof skillet over medium-high heat, and sear the stuffed chicken breasts for 2-3 minutes per side until browned.

6. Transfer the skillet to the preheated oven and bake for 15-20 minutes until chicken is cooked through.

7. Remove toothpicks before serving.

Nutritional Value (per serving):

- Calories: 290

- Protein: 34g

- Carbohydrates: 2g

- Fiber: 1g

- Fat: 15g

Recipe 48: Raspberry and Almond Butter Smoothie

Prep Time: 10 minutes Yields: 2 servings

Ingredients:

- 2 cups almond milk

- 2 cups frozen raspberries

- 2 tablespoons almond butter

- 1 banana

- 1 tablespoon honey

- 1/4 teaspoon almond extract (optional)

- Sliced almonds for garnish

Directions:

1. In a blender, combine almond milk, frozen raspberries, almond butter, banana, honey, and almond extract if using.

2. Blend until smooth and creamy.

3. Pour the smoothie into glasses and garnish with sliced almonds.

Nutritional Value (per serving):

- Calories: 230

- Protein: 4g

- Carbohydrates: 39g

- Fiber: 9g

- Fat: 9g

Recipe 49: Mediterranean Quinoa Bowl

Prep Time: 15 minutes Yields: 4 servings

Ingredients:

- 2 cups cooked quinoa

- 1 cup cucumber, diced

- 1 cup cherry tomatoes, halved

- 1/2 cup Kalamata olives, pitted and sliced

- 1/4 cup red onion, thinly sliced

- 1/4 cup crumbled feta cheese

- 2 tablespoons olive oil

- 2 tablespoons lemon juice

- Fresh oregano leaves for garnish

- Salt and pepper to taste

Directions:

1. In a bowl, combine cooked quinoa, diced cucumber, cherry tomatoes, sliced Kalamata olives, thinly sliced red onion, and crumbled feta cheese.

2. In a separate bowl, whisk together olive oil, lemon juice, salt, and pepper.

3. Drizzle the dressing over the quinoa salad and toss to combine.

4. Garnish with fresh oregano leaves before serving.

Nutritional Value (per serving):

- Calories: 290

- Protein: 7g

- Carbohydrates: 31g

- Fiber: 5g

- Fat: 16g

Recipe 50: Dark Chocolate and Berry Parfait

Prep Time: 10 minutes Yields: 2 servings

Ingredients:

- 1 cup Greek yogurt

- 1/2 cup mixed berries (strawberries, blueberries, raspberries)

- 2 tablespoons dark chocolate chips

- 2 tablespoons honey

- 1/4 cup granola

Directions:

1. In serving glasses, layer Greek yogurt, mixed berries, dark chocolate chips, honey, and granola.

2. Repeat the layers.

3. Finish with a drizzle of honey on top.

4. Serve immediately.

Nutritional Value (per serving):

- Calories: 330

- Protein: 13g

- Carbohydrates: 45g

- Fiber: 4g

- Fat: 12g

CONCLUSION

As we reach the end of "Brain-Boosting Recipes for Cognitive Wellness," we want to express our gratitude for joining us on this culinary journey. We hope you've not only discovered a treasure trove of delicious recipes but also gained a deeper understanding of the profound connection between food and cognitive health.

Cognitive wellness is a lifelong pursuit, and the choices we make in the kitchen can play a pivotal role in our mental vitality. With each meal you prepare from this cookbook, you've taken a step toward nurturing your mind and supporting your overall well-being.

We encourage you to continue exploring the world of brain-boosting ingredients and experimenting with new flavors and combinations. Cooking can be a joyful and therapeutic experience, and it's an opportunity to prioritize self-care and mental health.

Remember that nourishing your cognitive wellness is not just about what you eat but also how you eat. Savor your meals, share them with loved ones, and be present in each bite. Cultivate mindfulness around your food choices, and you'll find that the benefits extend beyond the plate.

We hope that these recipes have become a part of your culinary repertoire, enriching your daily life with flavors that delight your palate and nutrition that fuels your potential. Whether you're seeking improved focus, memory enhancement, or simply a well-rounded diet that supports your cognitive health, these recipes are here to serve as your guide.

As you continue on your journey toward cognitive wellness, remember that small, consistent steps can yield significant results. We encourage you to prioritize self-care, engage in regular physical activity, and practice mindfulness to complement the nourishing meals you enjoy.

Thank you for entrusting us with the opportunity to be a part of your quest for cognitive wellness. We believe that a healthy mind is the foundation for a fulfilling and vibrant life, and we hope that this cookbook has empowered you to take control of your mental well-being through the power of food.

Here's to a future filled with clarity, focus, and a zest for life. May your culinary adventures continue to inspire and invigorate you, allowing you to thrive in all aspects of your life.